Frusemide (Lasix)

A Clinician's Guide to Managing Hypertension and Edema with Water Pills

Asharani Sah

Frusemide (Lasix)

A Clinician's Guide to Managing Hypertension and Edema with Water Pills

Author: Asharani Sah

Published by: Self-Published
Publisher Address: Katihar, Bihar, India

First Edition

ISBN: 978-93-343-2541-6

This book is humbly dedicated to

Lord Shri Ramakrishna

Preface

Frusemide (Lasix) has long stood as one of the most indispensable drugs in the armamentarium of clinicians, particularly in the management of conditions characterized by fluid overload and acute hypertensive emergencies. Despite being widely used for decades, its clinical utility, potential hazards, and pharmacokinetic nuances often remain underappreciated in day-to-day medical practice.

This book, **"Frusemide (Lasix): A Clinician's Guide to Managing Hypertension and Edema with Water Pills,"** has been conceived with the aim of offering a clear, concise, and practical reference for doctors, paramedics, and healthcare professionals. It distills the essential pharmacology, clinical indications, dosing strategies, adverse effects, and monitoring protocols associated with this loop diuretic — and contextualizes its use across various patient populations and clinical scenarios.

Through structured chapters, the guide addresses:

- The historical background and development of loop diuretics
- Frusemide's mechanism of action and pharmacokinetics
- Its rational use in hypertension, heart failure, renal impairment, ascites, and special cases like hypercalcemia and raised intracranial pressure
- Practical dosing regimens tailored for different patient profiles, including pediatrics, geriatrics, pregnant women, and critically ill patients

- Drug interactions, contraindications, and combination therapies
- Real-world clinical cases offering prescribers a glimpse into practical challenges and effective solutions

In an era of increasing clinical complexity, rational diuretic therapy demands individualized patient care guided by pharmacology, pathophysiology, and patient-specific factors. It is hoped that this book will serve as a quick reference and educational resource for both early-career physicians and seasoned clinicians alike, enhancing confidence and precision in prescribing Frusemide safely and effectively.

I sincerely thank the many patients, colleagues, and medical mentors whose experiences, insights, and feedback shaped the practical wisdom contained within these pages.

May this guide contribute to safer, smarter, and more effective diuretic prescribing in everyday clinical practice.

Warm regards,

Asharani Sah
Author & Clinical Pharmacology Educator

Disclaimer

This book, Frusemide (Lasix): A Clinician's Guide to Managing Hypertension and Edema with Water Pills, is intended solely for educational and informational purposes for qualified healthcare professionals, including physicians, pharmacists, nurses, and other licensed medical practitioners.

The information contained herein is based on current scientific literature, clinical guidelines, regulatory approvals, and expert interpretation as of the time of publication. While every effort has been made to ensure accuracy and completeness, medical knowledge and treatment recommendations continue to evolve. Therefore, the author and publisher cannot guarantee that all information is up to date or free from errors or omissions.

*This publication is **not a substitute for clinical judgment** or institutional protocols, nor does it replace the need for consultation with appropriate medical authorities or pharmaceutical references. Prescribers are advised to refer to national and regional drug formularies, approved product labels, and clinical practice guidelines prior to making therapeutic decisions.*

The author and publisher disclaim any liability, loss, or damage incurred directly or indirectly as a result of the use or application of the information presented in this book. Inclusion of specific brands or trade names is for informational purposes only and does not imply endorsement.

Medical decisions must always be made in the context of the individual patient's condition and in consultation with appropriate clinical resources.

Table of Contents

Chapter 1: Introduction to Frusemide (Lasix)

Historical Overview and Development of Loop Diuretics

The management of fluid overload conditions such as edema, hypertension, and congestive heart failure has significantly evolved over the past century. Central to this progress has been the discovery and development of **loop diuretics**, a class of potent natriuretic agents that act on the renal tubular system to promote sodium and water excretion. Among these, **Frusemide (also known as Furosemide)** remains one of the most widely used and clinically significant drugs in modern medicine.

Early History of Diuretic Therapy

The use of diuretics can be traced back to ancient civilizations. Herbal preparations like **juniper berries** and **squill** were documented for their water-expelling effects as early as the Greco-Roman period. However, the modern pharmacological era began in the **early 20th century** with the development of inorganic mercurial diuretics such as **mercurial compounds (e.g., Mercuhydrin®)**, which were administered via injection for the treatment of edema and congestive heart failure. These agents, though effective, were associated with significant toxicity and cumbersome administration.

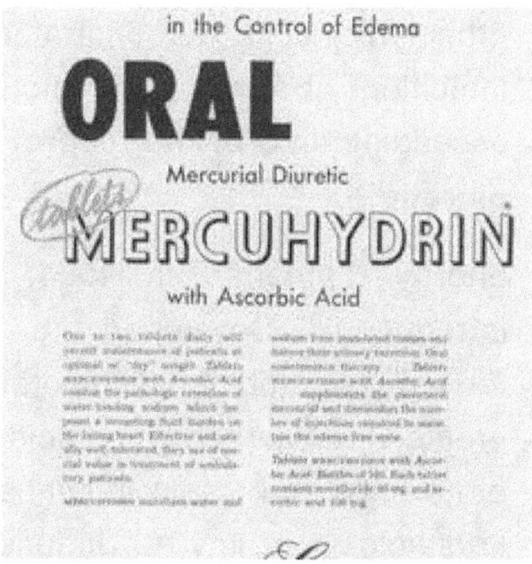

Discovery of Thiazide Diuretics

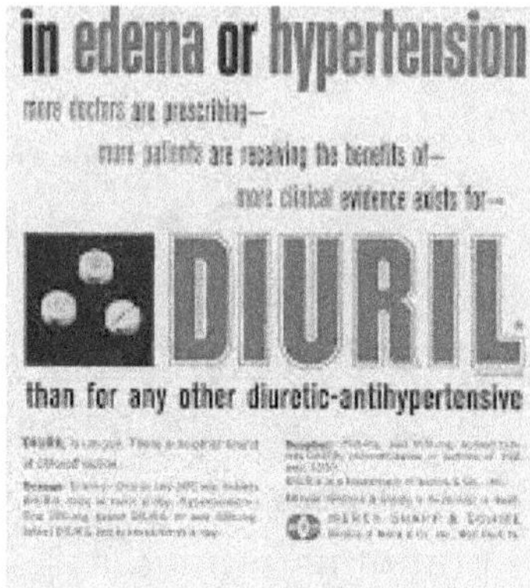

In the **1950s**, the development of **thiazide diuretics** marked a major advancement in diuretic therapy. **Chlorothiazide**, the first clinically available thiazide (brand name Diuril), offered oral administration and a safer side effect profile compared to mercurials. Thiazides became the preferred agents for managing mild to moderate hypertension and edema but were often insufficient in cases of severe fluid retention or advanced heart failure.

Emergence of Loop Diuretics

To address the limitations of thiazides in managing severe edema and acute volume overload, researchers pursued agents with more potent diuretic action. This led to the discovery of **ethacrynic acid** in **1962**, the first non-sulfonamide loop diuretic. Ethacrynic acid demonstrated powerful diuretic effects by inhibiting sodium and chloride reabsorption in the thick ascending limb of the loop of Henle — hence the term **'loop diuretic'**.

Shortly thereafter, in **1964**, **Frusemide (Furosemide)** was introduced. Developed by **Hoechst Pharmaceuticals**, Frusemide combined high potency with a more favourable safety profile than ethacrynic acid, which was associated with ototoxicity and gastrointestinal intolerance at higher doses. Frusemide's ability to induce rapid and profound diuresis revolutionized the management of acute pulmonary edema, severe congestive heart failure, nephrotic syndrome, and resistant hypertension.

Modern Loop Diuretics

Following Frusemide, other loop diuretics such as **bumetanide**, **torsemide**, and **azosemide** were introduced to clinical practice. These agents offer variations in potency, bioavailability, and duration of action, providing clinicians with valuable options to tailor therapy based on individual patient needs.

- **Bumetanide**: More potent than Frusemide, with a shorter half-life.
- **Torsemide**: Longer duration of action and higher oral bioavailability.
- **Ethacrynic acid**: Reserved for patients allergic to sulfonamide-based diuretics.

Current Relevance

From toxic mercury compounds to **targeted, life-saving drugs**, loop diuretics like frusemide represent a triumph of pharmacological innovation. Their history underscores the importance of **balancing efficacy with safety**—a lesson still relevant in today's precision medicine era.

Today, loop diuretics — particularly Frusemide — remain indispensable in clinical practice, forming the cornerstone of treatment for a wide range of conditions involving volume overload. Their pharmacological properties, rapid onset of action, and versatility in both oral and intravenous formulations have made them vital in both acute care and chronic disease management.

Ongoing research continues to refine loop diuretic use, exploring combination therapies, individualized dosing strategies, and the management of diuretic resistance, ensuring these agents maintain their essential role in modern therapeutics.

Chemical Structure and Pharmacological Class

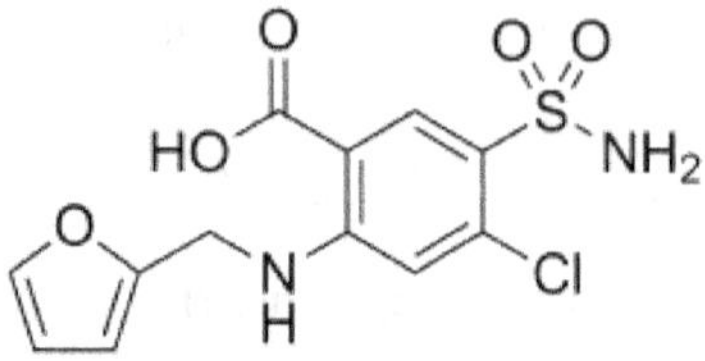

Frusemide is a **sulfonamide derivative** and structurally classified as an **aryloxyacetic acid.** Its chemical name is: **4-chloro-N-furfuryl-5-sulfamoylanthranilic acid.** The molecular formula is: **C12H11ClN2O5S.**

Frusemide is classified as a **loop diuretic** or **high-ceiling diuretic**. The term *high-ceiling* refers to the drug's ability to induce a profound increase in urinary sodium and water excretion — much higher than other classes like thiazides or potassium-sparing diuretics.

Classification Overview

Pharmacological Group	Example Drugs	Site of Action
Loop Diuretics (High-Ceiling)	Frusemide, Bumetanide, Torsemide, Ethacrynic acid	Thick ascending limb of loop of Henle
Thiazide Diuretics	Hydrochlorothiazide, Chlorthalidone	Distal convoluted tubule
Potassium-Sparing Diuretics	Spironolactone, Amiloride, Eplerenone	Collecting ducts
Osmotic Diuretics	Mannitol	Proximal tubule and loop of Henle
Carbonic Anhydrase Inhibitors	Acetazolamide	Proximal convoluted tubule

Clinical Correlations: How Structure Impacts Practice

A. Formulation Considerations

- **Oral vs. IV**:
    - Oral: Bioavailability varies (60–70%) due to **first-pass metabolism**.
    - IV: Bypasses gut → immediate effect (used in acute pulmonary edema).
- **Salt Forms**:
    - Frusemide is often formulated as a **sodium salt** to improve solubility.

B. Drug Interactions Rooted in Chemistry

- **NSAIDs (e.g., ibuprofen)**: Compete for renal secretion → reduce frusemide efficacy.
- Frusemide's sulfonamide structure aligns it chemically with certain thiazide diuretics and sulfonamide antibiotics, though their pharmacological targets differ. The presence of the sulfonamide group makes cross-reactivity with other sulfa drugs possible, an important consideration for clinicians managing patients with sulfonamide hypersensitivity.
- Among loop diuretics, Ethacrynic acid is unique as it lacks a sulfonamide group, making it an alternative in patients allergic to sulfa-containing diuretics.

Mechanism of Action — How Frusemide Works

Introduction

Frusemide (Furosemide) is a potent loop diuretic, widely regarded for its rapid and robust natriuretic and diuretic effects. Its primary mechanism involves inhibition of electrolyte reabsorption in the kidneys, specifically at a critical segment of the nephron. This chapter explains the precise pharmacological action of Frusemide, its renal site of activity, and the physiological consequences leading to diuresis and reduction of fluid overload.

Site of Action: Thick Ascending Limb of Loop of Henle

Frusemide acts predominantly on the **thick ascending limb (TAL) of the loop of Henle**, a crucial region in the nephron responsible for reabsorbing a significant portion of filtered sodium, chloride, and potassium.

The **TAL normally reabsorbs about 25–30% of filtered sodium and chloride** via a specific transport system called the:

Na^+-K^+-2Cl^- symporter (NKCC2)

This co-transporter moves **one sodium (Na^+), one potassium (K^+), and two chloride (Cl^-) ions** from the tubular lumen into the epithelial cells of the TAL.

How Frusemide Inhibits This Process

Frusemide binds to the chloride-binding site on the NKCC2 symporter, thereby inhibiting the reabsorption of sodium, potassium, and chloride. As a result:

- **Sodium and chloride remain in the tubular lumen** and are excreted in urine.

- **Potassium reabsorption is also reduced**, contributing to kaliuresis (loss of potassium in urine).
- The osmotic gradient created by retained electrolytes promotes **water excretion** (diuresis).

Secondary Physiological Effects

By disrupting the sodium reabsorption process in the TAL, Frusemide indirectly affects other physiological mechanisms:

- **Reduces medullary hypertonicity**: Decreased solute reabsorption lowers the concentration gradient needed for water reabsorption in the collecting duct.
- **Inhibits passive reabsorption of magnesium and calcium**: Normally driven by the positive luminal potential created by the NKCC2 symporter.
- **Activates the Renin-Angiotensin-Aldosterone System (RAAS)**: In response to decreased circulating volume, which can promote compensatory sodium and water retention downstream.
- **Causes vasodilation**: Frusemide promotes **renal prostaglandin synthesis**, which contributes to systemic and renal vasodilation, particularly beneficial in acute pulmonary edema.

Consequences of NKCC2 Inhibition

A. Hemodynamic Effects

- **Venodilation (IV frusemide):**
    - Occurs within minutes (before diuresis) due to **prostaglandin-mediated vasodilation.**
    - Useful in **acute pulmonary edema** for preload reduction.

B. Electrolyte and Fluid Excretion

Substance	Effect of Frusemide	Clinical Impact
Na^+	↑↑↑ Excretion (high efficacy)	Rapid diuresis; treats edema/HTN
Cl^-	↑↑↑ Excretion (parallels Na^+ loss)	Contributes to metabolic alkalosis
K^+	↑ Excretion (due to distal Na^+ delivery)	Risk of **hypokalemia**
Ca^{2+} & Mg^{2+}	↑ Excretion (unlike thiazides)	Risk of **hypocalcemia/hypomagnesemia**

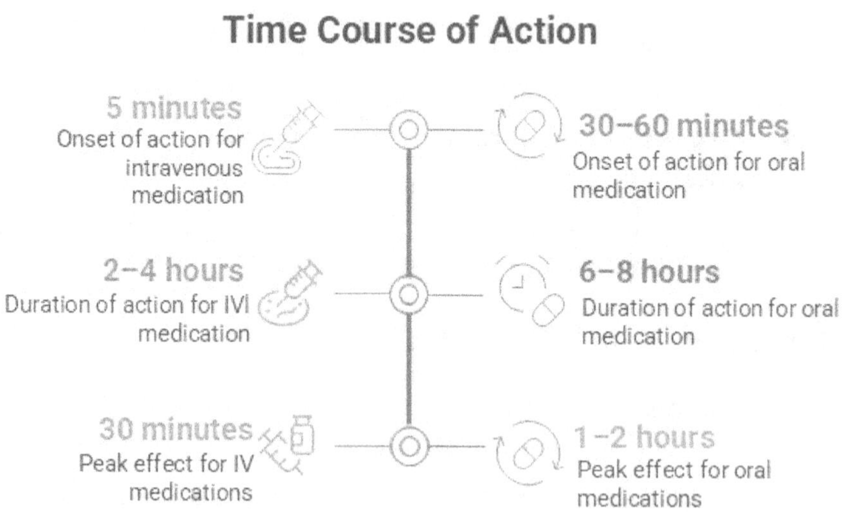

Summary of Mechanism

Action	Site/Effect
Inhibits **Na^+-K^+-$2Cl^-$ symporter**	Thick ascending limb of loop of Henle
↑ Sodium, chloride, potassium excretion	Increased diuresis and natriuresis
↓ Medullary hypertonicity	Impairs water reabsorption in collecting ducts
↑ Magnesium and calcium loss	Via reduced passive reabsorption
Activates RAAS	Due to volume depletion
Promotes vasodilation	Through renal prostaglandin synthesis

Clinical Implications

- Produces **rapid and powerful diuresis** ideal for acute pulmonary edema, severe edema, and resistant hypertension.
- Leads to **electrolyte disturbances**, including **hypokalemia**, **hyponatremia**, **hypocalcemia**, and **hypomagnesemia**, necessitating careful monitoring.
- Risk of **diuretic resistance** with prolonged use or in advanced renal failure due to compensatory mechanisms downstream in the nephron.

Frusemide remains a cornerstone of modern diuretic therapy owing to its well-defined and potent mechanism of action. By selectively inhibiting the Na^+-K^+-$2Cl^-$ symporter in the thick ascending limb, it efficiently addresses conditions of volume overload and hypertension, albeit with the need for diligent monitoring to avoid adverse effects.

Frusemide vs. Other Diuretics – A Comparative Guide for Clinicians

Diuretics are a diverse group of drugs classified based on their site and mechanism of action within the nephron. Each class differs in potency, duration, clinical indications, and adverse effect profiles. Understanding these differences is crucial for selecting the most appropriate agent for individual patient needs. So, this topic provides a **clinically oriented comparison** of frusemide with thiazides, potassium-sparing agents, osmotic diuretics, and other loop diuretics, focusing on **efficacy, safety, and optimal use cases**.

Pharmacological Comparison Table

Parameter	Loop Diuretics (Frusemide)	Thiazide Diuretics	Potassium-Sparing Diuretics	Osmotic Diuretics
Primary Site of Action	Thick ascending limb of loop of Henle	Distal convoluted tubule	Collecting duct	Proximal tubule & loop of Henle
Key Transporter Inhibited	Na^+-K^+-$2Cl^-$ symporter (NKCC2)	Na^+-Cl^- symporter	Epithelial sodium channels (ENaC) / Aldosterone receptor	Osmotic action
Potency (Natriuresis)	Very High	Moderate	Low	Variable
Onset of Action (Oral)	30–60 min	1–2 hours	2–4 hours	Rapid (IV)
Duration of Action	6–8 hours (oral)	12–18 hours	16–24 hours	4–6 hours
Effect on Potassium	Increases excretion (hypokalemia)	Increases excretion (hypokalemia)	Potassium-sparing	Minimal effect
Effect on Calcium	Increases excretion	Decreases excretion	Minimal effect	Minimal

Clinical Use	Acute pulmonary edema, CHF, nephrotic syndrome, severe edema, hypertension	Mild-moderate hypertension, mild edema	Adjunct in heart failure, cirrhosis, primary hyperaldosteronism	Cerebral edema, acute glaucoma, renal failure prevention
Risk of Electrolyte Imbalance	High	Moderate	Low	Low (but risk of fluid shifts)

Clinical Decision-Making: Choosing the Right Diuretic

A. Algorithm for Selection

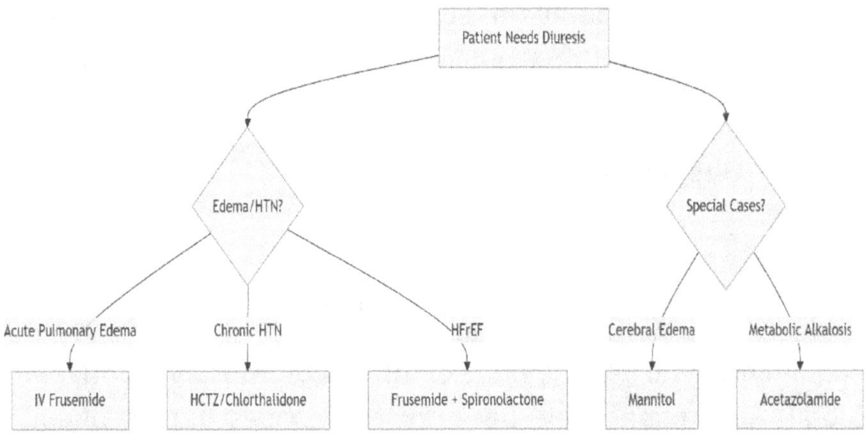

B. Avoiding Pitfalls

- **NSAIDs**: Reduce efficacy of **all diuretics except mannitol.**
- **Hypoalbuminemia**: Frusemide binds albumin → consider **albumin infusion** in cirrhosis.

Chapter 2: Pharmacokinetics and Pharmacodynamics

Absorption, Distribution, Metabolism, and Excretion (ADME)

Absorption

- **Frusemide is rapidly absorbed from the gastrointestinal tract** after oral administration.
- **Oral bioavailability** is highly variable, ranging from **10% to 90%** (average 50%).
- Food can **delay the absorption** and **reduce peak plasma concentrations** but typically does not alter the overall diuretic effect.
- **Onset of action**:
    - Oral: **30–60 minutes**
    - Intravenous (IV): **within 5 minutes**

Clinical Note: In conditions of **edema or intestinal congestion**, oral absorption may be impaired, necessitating parenteral administration for reliable effect.

Distribution

- **Plasma protein binding:** Frusemide is **highly protein-bound (~95%)**, primarily to **albumin**.
- It is **distributed widely in extracellular fluid compartments** but has limited penetration into intracellular spaces.

- The **volume of distribution (Vd)** is around **0.2 L/kg** in healthy adults.

Clinical Implication: In hypoalbuminemic states (e.g., nephrotic syndrome, liver cirrhosis), **free (active) drug levels increase**, potentially enhancing diuretic effect but also raising toxicity risk.

Metabolism

- Frusemide undergoes **minimal hepatic metabolism**.
- Approximately **10–20% of the drug is metabolized** in the liver to an inactive glucuronide conjugate.

Key Point: Since metabolism plays a minor role in its clearance, Frusemide can be safely used in patients with moderate liver dysfunction, although plasma protein binding may be altered.

Excretion

- **Primary route of elimination is renal excretion.**
- Around **80–90% of an administered dose is eliminated unchanged in the urine** via **active secretion in the proximal tubule** (through organic acid transporters).
- The remaining fraction is excreted via bile and feces.

Elimination half-life:

- **Healthy adults:** 1–2 hours
- **Prolonged in renal impairment** or congestive heart failure due to reduced renal perfusion.

Key Point: Frusemide requires **active secretion into the tubular lumen** to reach its site of action in the loop of Henle. In **severe renal failure or with competing drugs (e.g., NSAIDs,**

probenecid), this secretion is reduced, leading to diminished diuretic response.

Pharmacokinetic Summary Table

Parameter	Details
Absorption (Oral Bioavailability)	10–90% (average ~50%)
Time to Peak (Tmax)	Oral: 1–2 hours; IV: 30 min
Plasma Protein Binding	~95%
Volume of Distribution (Vd)	0.2 L/kg
Metabolism	~10–20% hepatic (glucuronidation)
Elimination Half-life	1–2 hours
Primary Excretion Route	Renal (80–90% unchanged)
Excretion Mechanism	Active tubular secretion

Clinical Implications

- **Reduced efficacy in hypoalbuminemia** due to impaired protein-bound transport to secretion sites.
- **Oral absorption variability** necessitates individualized dosing, particularly in edematous or critically ill patients.
- **Short half-life** favors flexible dosing but may necessitate multiple daily doses for sustained diuresis.
- **Competition for renal tubular secretion** (e.g., with NSAIDs) can impair Frusemide's delivery to its site of action, leading to **diuretic resistance**.

Onset and Duration of Action

Onset of Action

The **onset of action** refers to the time it takes for Frusemide to start producing a measurable diuretic effect after administration:

- **Oral administration:**
    - Onset typically occurs within **30–60 minutes**.
    - Slightly delayed when taken with food but without major loss in total diuretic effect.
- **Intravenous (IV) administration:**
    - Onset is rapid, occurring within **5 minutes**.
    - Highly useful in emergency settings like acute pulmonary edema or hypertensive crisis.
- **Intramuscular (IM) administration:**
    - Less preferred due to variable and unpredictable absorption.

Clinical Insight: In patients with compromised gut absorption (e.g., severe edema, gut hypoperfusion), IV Frusemide ensures predictable onset and therapeutic response.

Duration of Action

Duration reflects how long the drug continues exerting its clinical effect:

- **Oral administration:**
    - Lasts **6–8 hours**.
- **IV administration:**
    - Shorter, lasting around **2–4 hours**.

- **IM administration:**
    - Typically **4–6 hours**, though less predictable.

Key Consideration: The short half-life and relatively brief action mean that **multiple daily doses or continuous infusions** may be required in cases of severe edema or acute renal decompensation to maintain fluid control.

Dose-Response Relationship

Frusemide has a **non-linear, dose-dependent diuretic response**:

- **Lower doses (<20 mg IV or <40 mg oral)** may produce minimal diuresis in edematous or renal-impaired patients.
- **Higher doses increase both natriuresis and diuresis up to a ceiling dose** beyond which no further significant diuretic effect is achieved.
- This "ceiling effect" necessitates careful titration based on clinical needs.

Approximate Ceiling Doses:

- **Normal renal function:** 80–120 mg/day
- **Severe renal impairment:** 160–400 mg/day (higher ceiling due to reduced renal delivery)

Pharmacodynamic Summary Table

Parameter	Oral	IV
Onset of Action	30–60 minutes	5 minutes
Peak Effect	1–2 hours	30–60 minutes
Duration of Action	6–8 hours	2–4 hours
Ceiling Dose (approx.)	80–120 mg/day	160–400 mg/day (in renal failure)

Factors Affecting Drug Response (Age, Renal Function, Drug Interactions)

1 Age

◆ Neonates and Infants

- **Increased volume of distribution** and **immature renal tubular secretion** can prolong the half-life of Frusemide.
- Risk of **electrolyte imbalance and nephrocalcinosis** is higher in preterm and neonatal populations.

Clinical Note:
Use the lowest effective dose and monitor electrolytes closely.

◆ Elderly Patients

- **Reduced renal function** and **altered pharmacokinetics** lead to **enhanced diuretic sensitivity**.
- Higher risk of **postural hypotension, dehydration, and electrolyte disturbances**.
- Co-morbidities and polypharmacy increase the potential for adverse drug interactions.

Practice Tip:
Start at lower doses (e.g., 20 mg oral) and titrate cautiously with regular monitoring.

2 Renal Function

Frusemide relies on active tubular secretion to reach its site of action. In patients with **renal impairment**:

- Diuretic delivery to the tubular lumen decreases.
- Higher doses are required to achieve desired effects.
- The **ceiling dose increases** with declining renal function (up to 400–600 mg/day in advanced kidney disease).
- Risk of **ototoxicity and electrolyte derangements** is greater, especially at high IV doses.

Clinical Considerations:

- Avoid concurrent nephrotoxic agents (e.g., aminoglycosides).
- Use **higher but carefully titrated doses** in diuretic-resistant states.
- Consider combination diuretic therapy (e.g., with Metolazone or Spironolactone) in refractory edema.

3 Drug Interactions

Frusemide's pharmacokinetics and pharmacodynamics are influenced by several concomitant medications:

Interacting Drug/Category	Type of Interaction	Clinical Impact
Aminoglycosides (e.g., Gentamicin)	Additive ototoxicity	Risk of hearing loss, especially with high IV Frusemide doses
NSAIDs (e.g., Ibuprofen)	Reduced diuretic efficacy	By decreasing renal prostaglandin synthesis and renal blood flow
ACE Inhibitors / ARBs	Potentiation of hypotension and hyperkalemia	Monitor BP, electrolytes, especially when combined with potassium-sparing diuretics
Digitalis (Digoxin)	Increased risk of arrhythmias	Due to Frusemide-induced hypokalemia
Probenecid	Reduces tubular secretion of Frusemide	Decreases diuretic effect
Lithium	Reduced renal clearance of Lithium	Raises risk of lithium toxicity; requires close monitoring

Bioavailability and Formulations (IV vs. Oral)

Bioavailability Overview

Bioavailability refers to the proportion of an administered dose that reaches the systemic circulation in an active form.

- **Oral bioavailability of Frusemide is highly variable**, ranging from **10% to 90%**, with an average around **50%.**
- **Intravenous (IV) administration provides 100% bioavailability**, bypassing gastrointestinal absorption and first-pass metabolism.

Key Factors Affecting Oral Bioavailability:

- Presence of food (can delay absorption and reduce peak plasma concentration).
- Intestinal edema or congestion (reduces absorption in heart failure, liver cirrhosis, nephrotic syndrome).
- Variations in individual gut motility and perfusion.

Clinical Note:
In acute or severe conditions where rapid and reliable diuresis is needed, **IV administration is preferred**.

Frusemide Formulations

Formulation Type	Strengths Available	Common Uses
Oral Tablet	20 mg, 40 mg, 80 mg	Chronic management of edema, hypertension
Oral Solution	10 mg/mL, 40 mg/5 mL	Pediatric use, dysphagic or critically ill patients
Intravenous Injection	10 mg/mL (2 mL or 5 mL ampoules)	Emergency management of pulmonary edema, hypertensive crisis, severe edema

Chapter 3: Clinical Indications for Frusemide

Frusemide (Lasix) remains one of the most widely used loop diuretics in clinical medicine. Its ability to rapidly mobilize fluid makes it valuable in multiple conditions involving fluid overload and electrolyte imbalances. This chapter outlines the **approved and off-label clinical uses of Frusemide**, highlighting appropriate dosing strategies, preferred routes, and safety considerations.

Treatment of Hypertension: When and How to Use

While not a first-line antihypertensive, **Frusemide is valuable in specific scenarios:**

- **Severe Hypertension or Hypertensive Crisis** → **IV bolus (20–40 mg)** helps reduce intravascular volume and lower blood pressure rapidly.
- **Resistant Hypertension** → Added when BP remains uncontrolled despite optimal use of first-line drugs, particularly in:
    - **CKD patients with volume overload**
    - **Heart failure with hypertension**

Dosing:

- Oral: **20–80 mg/day**, titrated based on response.
- IV: For acute BP lowering — **20–40 mg IV**, repeat as needed.

Caution:
Avoid over-aggressive diuresis which can precipitate hypotension and electrolyte imbalance.

Management of Edema (Cardiac, Hepatic, Renal, and Pulmonary Causes)

Frusemide is the cornerstone drug for treating edema secondary to:

- **Cardiac Failure**
    - Relieves pulmonary and peripheral edema.
    - **Oral 20–80 mg/day** or **IV bolus in acute settings.**
- **Cirrhotic Ascites**
    - Given orally in combination with Spironolactone.
    - Start with **20–40 mg/day**, adjust cautiously to avoid electrolyte imbalance.
- **Nephrotic Syndrome**
    - High doses may be required due to hypoalbuminemia impairing diuretic delivery.
    - **Oral: 40–160 mg/day**; consider IV in resistant cases.
- **Pulmonary Edema**
    - Rapid IV Frusemide reduces venous return and pulmonary congestion.
    - **20–40 mg IV bolus**, repeat or double as needed.

Clinical Tip:
In edema-resistant states, combination with thiazides (e.g., Metolazone) may enhance natriuresis.

Acute and Chronic Heart Failure: Role of Frusemide

Frusemide is integral in both acute decompensated and stable chronic heart failure:

- **Acute Decompensated Heart Failure (ADHF)**
    - Rapid IV bolus reduces preload, pulmonary congestion.
    - Initial dose: **20–40 mg IV**, titrate based on clinical response and urine output.
- **Chronic Heart Failure**
    - Maintains euvolemia, relieves symptoms.
    - **Oral: 20–80 mg/day** in divided doses.
    - Dose escalation based on weight monitoring and edema control.

Monitoring:
Regular checks for hypokalemia, renal function, and over-diuresis.

Use in Nephrotic Syndrome and Renal Impairment

- **Nephrotic Syndrome**
    - Hypoalbuminemia reduces Frusemide efficacy.
    - Requires **higher doses (80–160 mg/day oral)** or **IV boluses.**
    - Combination with albumin infusions occasionally considered in severe cases.
- **Chronic Kidney Disease (CKD)**
    - Frusemide remains effective at high doses even in moderate-to-severe CKD.

- Dose adjustments:
  - GFR > 30 mL/min: **40–80 mg/day**
  - GFR < 30 mL/min: may require **160–400 mg/day**
- **Avoid combination with nephrotoxic agents.**

Practice Note:
In end-stage renal disease (ESRD), diuretic benefit is limited to urine-producing patients.

Special Cases: Ascites, Intracranial Hypertension, and Hypercalcemia

- **Ascites (due to Liver Cirrhosis)**
  - Combined with Spironolactone (usual ratio 100:40 mg).
  - **Initial Frusemide: 20–40 mg/day**, increased cautiously to avoid hepatorenal syndrome.
- **Intracranial Hypertension**
  - Used as adjunct with mannitol to lower raised intracranial pressure (ICP).
  - **IV 20–40 mg** given alongside osmotic diuretics in neurocritical care.
- **Hypercalcemia**
  - Enhances urinary calcium excretion.
  - After volume resuscitation, **IV Frusemide 20–40 mg every 2–4 hours**.
  - Monitor serum calcium, potassium, and magnesium closely.

Chapter 4: Dosing Strategies and Administration

Frusemide's dosing is highly individualized. Its diverse administration routes and dose flexibility allow clinicians to tailor therapy to a wide variety of clinical conditions, balancing efficacy with safety through careful monitoring.

Standard Dosing Guidelines for Different Conditions

Condition	Route	Starting Dose	Max/Adjusted Dose
Hypertension (oral)	Oral	20–40 mg once/twice daily	Up to 80 mg/day
Acute Pulmonary Edema	IV	20–40 mg IV bolus	Repeat or double every 2 hours as needed
Chronic Heart Failure	Oral	20–80 mg/day	Up to 320 mg/day (divided doses)
Nephrotic Syndrome	Oral/IV	40–160 mg/day	IV infusion or higher bolus doses
Ascites in Cirrhosis	Oral	20–40 mg/day	Up to 160 mg/day (with Spironolactone)
Hypercalcemia (IV)	IV	20–40 mg IV every 2–4 hrs	Adjust based on calcium levels
Raised ICP (with Mannitol)	IV	20–40 mg IV bolus	Based on ICP response

IV vs. Oral Administration: Pros and Cons

Parameter	IV Route	Oral Route
Bioavailability	100%	Variable (10–90%)
Onset of Action	5 minutes	30–60 minutes
Use in Emergencies	Ideal (pulmonary edema, hypertensive crisis)	Not preferred
Cost & Convenience	Higher cost, requires IV access	Cheaper, convenient for maintenance
Use in GI Edema	Effective despite gut congestion	Poor absorption in gut edema

Clinical Insight:
IV route preferred in acute, unstable conditions; switch to oral once stable.

Adjusting Doses in Renal and Hepatic Dysfunction

◆ **Renal Dysfunction**

- **Moderate CKD (GFR 30–60 mL/min):**
  Start with higher oral doses (**40–160 mg/day**).
- **Severe CKD (GFR <30 mL/min):**
  May require **up to 400–600 mg/day** orally or as IV infusion.

Key Point:
Ceiling dose increases with declining renal function.

◆ **Hepatic Impairment (Cirrhosis & Ascites)**

- Start low: **20–40 mg/day**
- Increase cautiously, monitor electrolytes and renal function.
- Combine with Spironolactone to prevent hypokalemia and natriuresis resistance.

Warning:
Rapid diuresis may trigger **hepatorenal syndrome**.

Continuous Infusion vs. Bolus Dosing in Critical Care

Dosing Method	Advantages	Disadvantages
IV Bolus	Simple, rapid effect	Risk of post-diuretic sodium retention, variable peaks and troughs
Continuous IV Infusion	Steady diuresis, lower total dose, reduced ototoxicity risk	Requires infusion pump, monitoring

Typical Infusion Dose:

- Start with **2–4 mg/hour IV,** titrate based on urine output.

Preferred in:

- **Acute decompensated heart failure**
- **Resistant edema in ICU**
- **Severe CKD with fluid overload**

Pediatric and Geriatric Considerations

Pediatric Use

- **Neonates/Infants:**
  - Oral: **1–2 mg/kg/dose** every 12–24 hours
  - IV: **0.5–1 mg/kg/dose**, may repeat after 6–8 hours
- **Children:**
  - Oral: **1–2 mg/kg/day** in 1–2 divided doses

Caution:
Higher risk of electrolyte imbalance, nephrocalcinosis.

Geriatric Use

- Start at lower doses: **20 mg/day orally**
- Titrate slowly based on BP, weight, edema
- **Monitor closely for hypotension, electrolyte imbalance, and renal dysfunction**

Key Practice Tip:
In elderly patients, avoid rapid fluid shifts to prevent falls, syncope, and cognitive disturbances.

Chapter 5: Adverse Effects and Monitoring

Common Side Effects

◆ Electrolyte Imbalances

Frusemide increases urinary excretion of several electrolytes:

- **Hypokalemia** (most frequent)
- **Hyponatremia**
- **Hypocalcemia**
- **Hypomagnesemia**

Clinical Signs:
Muscle cramps, fatigue, arrhythmias, altered sensorium.

Management:

- Regular electrolyte monitoring
- Potassium supplementation or potassium-sparing diuretic (Spironolactone)
- IV electrolyte correction in severe cases

◆ Dehydration

Excessive diuresis can lead to:

- Hypovolemia
- Dry mucous membranes
- Postural hypotension
- Acute kidney injury

Management:
Adjust dose based on weight, BP, and urine output. Provide IV fluids if hypovolemia occurs.

◆ Ototoxicity

High-dose IV Frusemide can cause reversible or irreversible hearing loss, especially when:

- Given too rapidly (>4 mg/min)
- Combined with other ototoxic drugs (e.g., aminoglycosides)

Prevention:
Slow IV administration and monitoring hearing status during high-dose therapy.

Rare but Serious Complications

- **Severe Hypotension:**
  Especially in elderly, volume-depleted, or over-diuresed patients.
- **Allergic Reactions:**
  Urticaria, rash, or rare anaphylaxis, especially in patients with sulfa allergy.
- **Pancreatitis:**
  Rare idiosyncratic reaction — presents with abdominal pain, elevated amylase/lipase.
- **Thromboembolism:**
  From rapid hemoconcentration in aggressive diuresis.

Management:
Immediate cessation of drug in severe reactions and supportive care.

Monitoring Parameters

Parameter	Frequency	Why Monitor?
Serum Potassium, Sodium, Magnesium, Calcium	Baseline, then 1–2 times weekly (acute use)	Detect electrolyte imbalances
Renal Function (Serum Creatinine, eGFR)	Baseline, 2–3 days after initiation or dose change	Prevent acute kidney injury
Fluid Balance (Weight, Input-Output Chart)	Daily (hospitalized); weekly (OPD)	Guide diuretic dosing and prevent over/under-diuresis
Blood Pressure (lying & standing)	Daily or every shift in hospital	Detect hypotension
Hearing Assessment (high-dose IV use)	Periodically if ototoxic risk	Early detection of ototoxicity

Managing Diuretic Resistance

Diuretic resistance occurs when expected natriuresis is not achieved despite adequate dosing.

Causes:

- Intestinal edema impairing oral absorption
- Excessive sodium intake
- Nephrotic syndrome with low albumin
- Renal dysfunction
- Rebound sodium retention after bolus dosing

Management Strategies:

- **Switch to or combine with IV continuous infusion**
- **Use of sequential nephron blockade**: add Thiazide (e.g., Metolazone)
- **Sodium restriction** (<2 g/day)
- **Optimize renal perfusion**: cautious fluid management
- **Add albumin infusion (in hypoalbuminemic states)** to improve diuretic delivery

Practical Tip:
Monitor urine output hourly in resistant cases, and adjust therapy promptly.

Chapter 6: Drug Interactions and Contraindications

Major Drug Interactions

Interacting Drug/Class	Effect on Frusemide or Patient	Clinical Consequence
NSAIDs (e.g., Ibuprofen, Diclofenac)	Blunt diuretic and antihypertensive effects by reducing renal prostaglandin synthesis	Reduced natriuresis, risk of fluid overload
ACE Inhibitors/ARBs (e.g., Enalapril, Losartan)	Risk of profound hypotension and acute kidney injury when combined in volume-depleted patients	Monitor BP and renal function closely; start ACEi after stabilizing volume
Digoxin	Hypokalemia from Frusemide enhances Digoxin toxicity (arrhythmias)	Monitor potassium; correct before starting Digoxin
Aminoglycosides (e.g., Gentamicin)	Increased risk of ototoxicity and nephrotoxicity when used concurrently	Avoid high-dose combinations; use cautiously if necessary
Lithium	Frusemide reduces renal clearance of lithium, increasing risk of lithium toxicity	Regularly monitor lithium levels; adjust dose accordingly
Corticosteroids	Additive risk of hypokalemia	Monitor potassium; supplement if needed
Antidiabetic agents	Frusemide-induced hyperglycemia may blunt antidiabetic effects	Monitor blood glucose in diabetics on diuretics

Contraindications and Precautions

Absolute Contraindications:

- **Anuria (no urine output)** not responsive to trial diuresis
- **Severe electrolyte depletion** (e.g., hypokalemia, hyponatremia)
- **Allergy to Frusemide or sulfa-containing drugs**

Relative Contraindications (Use Cautiously):

- **Hepatic coma** (risk of precipitating encephalopathy)
- **Severe hyponatremia or hypokalemia**
- **Gout** (may raise serum uric acid levels)
- **Pregnancy and lactation** (see Chapter 7)
- **Hypovolemia or hypotension**

Precautions:

- Monitor for rapid shifts in electrolytes and intravascular volume.
- Titrate doses slowly in elderly and patients with renal/hepatic dysfunction.
- Avoid overzealous diuresis in heart failure or cirrhosis patients to prevent complications like hepatorenal syndrome.

Clinical Insight:
Even in contraindicated cases, temporary Frusemide use may be lifesaving in emergencies (e.g., pulmonary edema) — benefits should be weighed against risks.

Combination Therapy with Other Diuretics

Why Combine Diuretics?

- Overcome **diuretic resistance**
- Synergistic action on different nephron sites

Common Diuretic Combinations:

Frusemide +	Site of Action	Clinical Use
Thiazides (e.g., Metolazone, Hydrochlorothiazide)	Distal convoluted tubule	Resistant edema, severe CHF, CKD
Spironolactone	Collecting duct (aldosterone antagonist)	Cirrhosis-related ascites, CHF, hypokalemia prevention
Amiloride	Collecting duct (ENaC blocker)	Hypokalemia prevention with high-dose Frusemide
Mannitol	Proximal tubule and descending loop	Raised intracranial pressure, acute renal failure (with Frusemide to enhance effect)

Important Points:

- Monitor electrolytes vigilantly when combining diuretics, particularly for **hypokalemia, hyponatremia, and hypovolemia**
- Sequential nephron blockade (Frusemide + Thiazide) highly effective in resistant edema but carries increased risk of severe electrolyte imbalance
- Frusemide with Spironolactone is a standard strategy in **cirrhotic ascites management**

Example Regimen:
Frusemide 40 mg + Spironolactone 100 mg is a typical starting ratio in cirrhotic ascites.

Clinical Tip:
When adding a second diuretic, start with a low dose and titrate cautiously under close monitoring.

Frusemide interacts with several essential drug classes, demanding careful medication reconciliation and monitoring to prevent adverse outcomes. Its strategic combination with other diuretics can enhance therapeutic efficacy, especially in refractory edema, but must be balanced against the risk of electrolyte and volume disturbances.

Chapter 7: Special Populations and Clinical Scenarios

Frusemide is a vital medication in diverse clinical scenarios. Its application in special populations — like pregnant women, critically ill patients, perioperative cases, and chronic users — requires individualized assessment, cautious dosing, and vigilant monitoring to ensure both safety and efficacy.

Use in Pregnancy and Lactation

Pregnancy:

- **FDA Category C**: Animal studies have shown adverse fetal effects, but no controlled human studies exist.
- Generally **avoided in uncomplicated pregnancy** due to risk of:
  - Fetal growth restriction
  - Electrolyte imbalance in the fetus
  - Reduced placental perfusion

Indications in Pregnancy:

- Acute pulmonary edema (e.g., preeclampsia with fluid overload)
- Severe heart failure during pregnancy
- Rarely for resistant hypertension as a third-line agent

Dosing:
Start low — **20 mg IV/Oral**; titrate cautiously with continuous maternal and fetal monitoring.

Lactation:

- Frusemide is excreted in breast milk.
- May **suppress lactation** at high doses.
- **Use cautiously**; if essential, monitor infant for signs of dehydration and poor weight gain.

Frusemide in Critical Care and Emergency Medicine

Frusemide is a first-line agent in acute care for:

- **Acute decompensated heart failure**
- **Pulmonary edema**
- **Hypertensive crisis with fluid overload**
- **Acute hypercalcemia**
- **Raised intracranial pressure (with mannitol)**

Dosing Approach:

- **IV Bolus:** 20–40 mg; repeat/double every 2 hours as needed

- **Continuous IV Infusion:** 2–4 mg/hour, titrated based on urine output and hemodynamics

Critical Considerations:

- Rapid BP changes can destabilize patients

- Monitor electrolytes, renal function, fluid status hourly in ICU settings

- Use in combination with vasodilators and inotropes as appropriate

Practical Tip:
In massive pulmonary edema, an **initial IV push followed by infusion** is more effective than repeated boluses alone.

Perioperative and Anesthetic Considerations

Preoperative:

- Continue diuretics in patients with severe heart failure, pulmonary edema, or fluid overload
- Hold if patient is volume-depleted or hypotensive

Intraoperative:

- Used intraoperatively to manage:
  - Oliguria during surgery
  - Pulmonary edema
  - Elevated intracranial pressure

Anesthetic Interactions:

- Potentiates hypotension under general anesthesia
- Risk of electrolyte disturbances affecting neuromuscular blocking agents (prolonged action of non-depolarizing agents)

Postoperative:

- Resume carefully once euvolemia is ensured
- Monitor closely for hypokalemia, hypovolemia, and AKI, especially if nephrotoxic drugs were used perioperatively

Long-Term Use vs. Short-Term Therapy

Parameter	Short-Term Use	Long-Term Use
Common Indications	Pulmonary edema, hypertensive emergencies, acute decompensated heart failure	Chronic heart failure, cirrhotic ascites, CKD-related edema
Dosing Strategy	IV bolus/infusion; rapid effect	Oral maintenance dosing; adjusted based on weight and symptoms
Risks	Electrolyte imbalance, hypovolemia, AKI, ototoxicity	Chronic hypokalemia, hyperuricemia, glucose intolerance, diuretic resistance
Monitoring Needs	Frequent vitals, electrolytes, renal function, fluid balance	Regular monitoring of weight, electrolytes, renal function, BP
Clinical Caution	Avoid over-diuresis; titrate based on rapid clinical response	Periodic reassessment of indication, minimizing chronic high-dose exposure

Practical Insight:

- **Long-term Frusemide use requires periodic drug holidays** or dose tapering to prevent diuretic resistance and minimize long-term metabolic effects.
- Always re-evaluate the continued need for Frusemide in stable patients.

Chapter 8: Case Studies and Clinical Pearls

The following cases illustrate practical challenges and evidence-based strategies for optimizing Frusemide therapy in complex clinical scenarios. Tailoring dose, route, and combination regimens — while monitoring electrolytes, renal function, and hemodynamics — ensures both therapeutic efficacy and patient safety.

Case 1: Acute Pulmonary Edema in Heart Failure

Patient Profile:

65-year-old male with a history of **ischemic cardiomyopathy (EF 30%)**, presenting with acute breathlessness, orthopnea, and pink frothy sputum.

Examination:

- BP: 150/90 mmHg
- HR: 110/min
- SpO_2: 84% on room air
- Bilateral basal crepitations

Investigations:

- CXR: Pulmonary congestion
- BNP: 1120 pg/mL
- Serum creatinine: 1.2 mg/dL

Management:

- **Oxygen by face mask**

- **IV Frusemide 40 mg bolus**, followed by 40 mg IV 6 hourly
- Nitrates infusion for afterload reduction
- Low-dose inotropes started for hypotension risk
- Monitoring of urine output, electrolytes, and BP hourly

Outcome:

- Significant clinical improvement within 6 hours
- Shifted to oral Frusemide 40 mg twice daily after stabilization

Clinical Pearl:
In acute pulmonary edema, IV Frusemide acts rapidly to reduce preload, but must be balanced with hemodynamic monitoring to avoid hypotension and renal hypoperfusion.

Case 2: Refractory Hypertension with Renal Impairment

Patient Profile:
58-year-old woman with **CKD stage 3 (eGFR 35 mL/min)**, uncontrolled hypertension on triple-drug therapy (Amlodipine, Losartan, and Hydrochlorothiazide).

Examination:

- BP: 180/100 mmHg
- No pedal edema
- Normal cardiovascular and respiratory findings

Investigations:

- Serum creatinine: 2.0 mg/dL

- Serum potassium: 4.5 mEq/L

Management:

- Stopped Hydrochlorothiazide due to reduced efficacy at eGFR <40 mL/min
- Initiated **Frusemide 80 mg/day orally** in divided doses
- Advised low-sodium diet and restricted fluid intake
- Continued ACE inhibitor cautiously with renal function monitoring

Outcome:

- BP reduced to 140/90 mmHg over 1 week
- Maintained good urine output without electrolyte imbalance

Clinical Pearl:
In CKD, Thiazide diuretics lose efficacy as GFR declines, while Frusemide remains effective at higher doses and can aid BP control and fluid balance.

Case 3: Diuretic Resistance in Nephrotic Syndrome

Patient Profile:
35-year-old male with **primary nephrotic syndrome** (albumin 2.0 g/dL), on Frusemide 160 mg/day with inadequate response.

Examination:

- BP: 130/80 mmHg
- Anasarca

- Urine output: <500 mL/day

Investigations:

- Serum creatinine: 1.3 mg/dL
- Serum albumin: 2.0 g/dL
- Sodium: 136 mEq/L
- Potassium: 3.8 mEq/L

Management:

- Administered **IV albumin 20% (100 mL)** over 4 hours
- Followed by **IV Frusemide 80 mg bolus**
- Added **Metolazone 2.5 mg once daily**
- Sodium restriction <2 g/day

Outcome:

- Urine output improved to 2 liters/day
- Weight reduction by 4 kg over 3 days
- Edema subsided over a week

Clinical Pearl:
In nephrotic syndrome, hypoalbuminemia impairs Frusemide delivery to the renal tubule. Combination with albumin or sequential nephron blockade enhances diuretic response.

Case 4: Electrolyte Imbalance in an Elderly Patient

Patient Profile:

78-year-old male with **congestive heart failure**, on chronic Frusemide 80 mg/day and Digoxin.

Examination:

- BP: 130/80 mmHg
- HR: 48/min (irregular)
- Confused, with mild dehydration signs

Investigations:

- Serum potassium: 2.8 mEq/L
- Serum sodium: 128 mEq/L
- ECG: Premature ventricular complexes (PVCs)
- Serum Digoxin: Elevated at 2.5 ng/mL

Management:

- Stopped Digoxin temporarily
- IV potassium chloride correction
- Reduced Frusemide to 40 mg/day
- Added **Spironolactone 25 mg/day**
- Monitored serum electrolytes and ECG daily

Outcome:

- Electrolytes normalized over 48 hours
- No further arrhythmias
- Cognitive status improved

Clinical Pearl:

Chronic high-dose Frusemide use in the elderly requires vigilant electrolyte and renal function monitoring. Hypokalemia potentiates Digoxin toxicity, increasing arrhythmia risk.

Chapter 9: Common Prescribing Errors and How to Avoid Them

Dosing Mistakes

Common Errors:

- **Using fixed, low oral doses (e.g., 20 mg/day) in advanced heart failure or renal dysfunction**, resulting in inadequate diuresis.
- **Rapid IV bolus dosing (>4 mg/min)** increasing risk of ototoxicity.
- **Failing to adjust doses based on renal function, body weight, and clinical response.**
- **Using Thiazide diuretics instead of loop diuretics** in advanced CKD where they're ineffective.

Prevention Strategies:

- Always tailor the dose to **disease severity and renal function**.
- Use **continuous infusions or higher ceiling doses** in resistant cases (especially CKD, nephrotic syndrome).
- Adhere to safe IV administration rates.
- Avoid "one-size-fits-all" dosing — reassess frequently.

Inadequate Monitoring

Common Errors:

- **Not checking serum electrolytes (K^+, Na^+, Mg^{2+}) regularly**, especially in high-risk or elderly patients.

- **Ignoring daily weight monitoring in edema management.**
- **Infrequent renal function assessment during high-dose or long-term use.**
- **Lack of urine output tracking in critical care settings.**

Prevention Strategies:

- Establish a **baseline renal panel and electrolytes** before initiating Frusemide.
- Monitor **weight daily**, particularly in heart failure and nephrotic syndrome.
- Check **serum electrolytes and creatinine** 48–72 hours after dose changes or IV initiation.
- Monitor **urine output hourly** in ICU or acute decompensated cases.

Misinterpretation of Symptoms

Common Errors:

- **Attributing hypotension, weakness, or confusion in elderly patients to age alone**, overlooking over-diuresis or electrolyte imbalance.
- **Missing early signs of hypokalemia** (fatigue, palpitations, cramps) until complications like arrhythmias occur.
- **Mistaking diuretic-induced postural hypotension for autonomic dysfunction.**

Prevention Strategies:

- Maintain a high index of suspicion for **Frusemide-related adverse effects** in any symptomatic patient on diuretics.
- Regularly assess **postural BP, cognitive status, and ECG** in at-risk groups.
- Educate patients on recognizing early signs of **electrolyte imbalance and dehydration**.

Preventing Drug Interactions

Common Errors:

- **Concurrent use of NSAIDs** without awareness of their antagonistic effect on diuretic action.
- **Combining Digoxin without correcting hypokalemia**, risking toxicity.
- **Co-prescribing other ototoxic drugs (e.g., Aminoglycosides) with IV Frusemide** at high doses.
- **Neglecting lithium level monitoring** in patients on Frusemide.

Prevention Strategies:

- Always **review concurrent medications** for potential interactions.
- Prefer **paracetamol over NSAIDs** for analgesia in volume-overloaded patients.
- Ensure **serum potassium ≥ 4.0 mEq/L** before starting Digoxin.

- Avoid combining multiple ototoxic agents or, if unavoidable, use the lowest effective doses with close monitoring.

Avoiding Overuse and Underuse

Common Errors:

- **Unnecessary prolonged Frusemide use** in patients with resolved edema, risking chronic electrolyte disturbances.
- **Failure to escalate doses or switch to combination diuretic therapy** in resistant cases.
- **Chronic low-dose therapy without reassessing ongoing need** in stable heart failure or post-decongestion phase.
- **Over-aggressive diuresis** causing hypovolemia, AKI, and hypotension.

Prevention Strategies:

- **Reassess indication for Frusemide regularly**, especially in chronic users.
- Adjust dosing based on **clinical response, weight, and fluid status** — avoid excessive diuresis.
- In resistant edema, consider **sequential nephron blockade** (e.g., adding Metolazone) rather than uncritically escalating Frusemide alone.
- Educate patients about **daily weight monitoring** and when to report symptoms of over or under-diuresis.

Chapter 10: Patient Counseling Essentials

Good patient counseling empowers individuals to participate actively in their care, prevents complications, and enhances adherence. Clear, personalized advice on **medication use, symptom recognition, diet, and monitoring** is essential for safe and successful Frusemide therapy.

Key Points for Patient Education

- Explain **why the medication is prescribed** — whether for edema, hypertension, heart failure, or another condition.
- Inform that it's a **diuretic (water pill)** designed to help remove excess salt and water from the body.
- Emphasize the importance of **regular blood tests** to monitor electrolytes and kidney function.
- Advise on **daily weight monitoring**, particularly in patients with heart failure or ascites.
- Encourage patients to **never adjust the dose or stop the medication without consulting their doctor.**
- Highlight potential **side effects** like dizziness, increased urination, muscle cramps, and weakness.

Example statement:

"This medicine helps your body get rid of extra salt and water through urine. It will make you pass urine more often. It's important you keep track of your weight and get regular blood tests while using this medication."

When and How to Take the Medication

- **Best taken in the morning** to avoid frequent nighttime urination.
- If a second dose is prescribed, advise taking it **before 4 PM**.
- Frusemide can be taken **with or without food**, but may cause less stomach upset if taken after meals.
- Ensure patients understand **not to double up on missed doses** — if forgotten, skip and take the next scheduled dose.
- Advise patients to **avoid alcohol** while on Frusemide, as it can worsen dizziness and dehydration.

Practical Tip:

For elderly or high-risk patients, ensure safe access to toilet facilities due to the rapid onset of diuresis.

Recognizing Warning Symptoms

Patients should be counseled to promptly report any of the following symptoms:

- **Excessive weakness, dizziness, or fainting spells**
- **Muscle cramps, palpitations, or irregular heartbeat**
- **Sudden weight gain or loss of more than 2 kg in 2–3 days**
- **Confusion, lethargy, or decreased urine output**
- **Signs of dehydration** — dry mouth, decreased skin turgor, reduced urination
- **Hearing disturbances** (especially with IV use)

Encourage patients to keep a **symptom diary** if possible for easier review during follow-ups.

Dietary Advice and Fluid Management

Sodium Restriction:

- Advise patients to limit **salt intake** as excess sodium counteracts the effect of Frusemide.
- Recommend avoiding processed, canned, and packaged foods high in sodium.
- Encourage use of **herbs and spices** instead of table salt.

Potassium Management:

- Explain that Frusemide may lower potassium levels.
- Depending on serum potassium and concurrent medications:
    - **Increase potassium-rich foods** (bananas, oranges, coconut water, spinach) if hypokalemic.
    - Or avoid excessive potassium intake if also on potassium-sparing diuretics.

Fluid Management:

- Instruct patients to follow **fluid restriction** if prescribed — especially in heart failure or severe edema.
- Educate about monitoring **urine output and daily weight**.
- Clarify that patients should avoid excessive fluid intake just because they are urinating more.

Example Advice:

"Reduce your salt use while cooking, avoid pickles and packaged snacks, and weigh yourself daily in the morning after emptying your bladder. If you suddenly gain 2 kg in 2 days, contact your doctor immediately."

www.ingramcontent.com/pod-product-compliance
Lightning Source LLC
Chambersburg PA
CBHW071521180726
48282CB00058B/785
9789334325416